UNDERSTANDING

SOUND

THERAPY

Unlock The Healing Power Of Sound For Targeting Wellness, Focus, Practical Applications, Key Insights And Techniques For Vibrant Living And More

DR. KARSON BRYAN

1

DISCLAIMER

This book's content is meant to be used solely for general informative purposes. Despite having taken every precaution to guarantee the content's accuracy, the author disclaims all duty and responsibility for any errors or omissions. It is recommended that readers exercise caution and, if needed, seek expert guidance. Any and all liability for losses, damages, or other outcomes arising from the use of the material included in this book is disclaimed by the author and publisher. All referenced product names and trademarks are the property of their respective owners and are merely cited for identification. Any likeness to real people or things is entirely accidental. Since it is a work of fiction, this book should not be used as a substitute for professional, legal, or medical advice. It is advised that readers seek advice on particular issues from qualified experts."

Please make sure that this disclaimer is modified to fit the particular requirements and subject matter of your book. Seeking advice from a legal expert is also a smart option if you have any questions or require a more thorough disclaimer for your specific book.

TABLE OF CONTENTS

CHAPTER ONE

SOUND THERAPY

INTRODUCTION

Utilizing the power of sound and vibration to enhance mental, emotional, and spiritual well-being, sound therapy is a holistic approach to healing. This therapeutic approach has a long history and is based on the idea that music has a profound effect on both the body and the mind. We will examine the foundational ideas of sound therapy in this introduction, as well as its historical development, scientific foundations, and the numerous advantages it provides to individuals seeking its calming and transforming effects.

WHAT IS SONOROUS TREATMENT?

A complementary and alternative therapy, sound therapy also called sound healing uses different sound frequencies, vibrations, and rhythms to help the body regain harmony and balance. The main idea is that our bodies are made of more than just physical stuff; they also have an energy and vibrational component. The idea behind sound therapy is that certain sounds and frequencies have the power to affect these energies, hence assisting in the correction of emotional and physical imbalances.

Sound therapy practitioners use a variety of tools and methods, such as gongs, singing bowls, tuning forks, chanting, and even recorded music created especially for therapeutic reasons. To remove blockages, lessen tension, encourage relaxation, and aid in healing, these instruments produce sound waves that resonate with the body's energy centers, or chakras, as well as various bodily parts.

THE HISTORY AND FOUNDATIONS OF SOUND HEALING

The origins of sound therapy can be found in ancient cultures, where music and sound played a crucial role in spiritual and therapeutic rites. Chants, drums, and other instruments were used by indigenous tribes all over the world to heal mental and physical illnesses as well as to establish a spiritual connection. Modern sound therapy has its roots in the Ayurvedic treatment of ancient India when voice toning and mantras were used.

These antiquated customs inspire the modern field of sound therapy, which blends them with cutting-edge knowledge and methods. Its increasing appeal as a supplemental therapeutic modality in recent decades has aided in its continued development and expansion.

THE SCIENTIFIC BASIS OF SOUND HEALING

The effectiveness of sound therapy is being supported by an increasing amount of scientific study, meaning that it is not just reliant on esoteric beliefs. Resonance and entrainment are the foundational concepts of sound therapy. When an external sound's vibrational frequency coincides with that of a particular bodily component, resonance takes place, intensifying the resonance and possibly even fostering healing.

The process through which one vibrating or rhythmic system aligns its frequency with another is known as entrainment. Entrainment is a common technique in sound treatment to assist in synchronizing the body's natural rhythms, which include breathing, heart rate, and brainwave patterns. According to studies, sound therapy helps lessen pain, stress, and anxiety. As a result, it is being utilized more often in clinical settings as an adjunct to conventional medical therapies.

THE ADVANTAGES OF SOUND THERAPY

Sound therapy has numerous advantages that touch on many facets of well-being. For relaxation, stress relief, anxiety relief, and sleep disorder relief, many resort to sound therapy. Deep relaxation brought on by sound treatments may speed up the healing process and improve general health.

Additionally, studies have shown that sound therapy enhances psychological and emotional health. It can be a technique for trauma and unprocessed emotions to be processed and released, promoting self-awareness and personal development. It can also improve creativity, focus, and cognitive function.

Sound therapy is a well-established therapeutic approach with a long history that is based on both conventional wisdom and cutting-edge research. It addresses the psychological, spiritual, and bodily facets of well-being and has a wide range of possible advantages. We will examine sound therapy's methods, tools, and particular uses as we go deeper into the field, giving you a thorough grasp of this amazing therapeutic strategy.

CHAPTER TWO

VIBRATION AND THE HUMAN FORM

THE EFFECTS OF SOUND ON THE BODY

A vital component of life, sound has a wide range of deep-seated effects on the human body. Sound can elicit a range of emotions, affect our moods, and even have an effect on our physical health. Sound stimulates the auditory system, which is one of the most direct ways that sound impacts the body. The eardrum vibrates as sound waves enter the ear and pass through the ear canal. The microscopic hair cells in the inner ear then receive these vibrations and transform them into electrical impulses that the brain may perceive as sound. This is a sensory experience that affects more than just the auditory system; it sets off a series of bodily reactions.

Sound has an impact on the body that goes beyond the sense of hearing. A relaxation reaction to certain sounds can lower heart rate, ease tension, and lessen anxiety. On the other hand, startling and loud noises can set off the body's fight-or-flight reaction, which raises heart rate and attentiveness. Specifically, music has a strong emotional impact on us and can be used therapeutically to elevate mood and enhance mental health. Music's ability to synchronize brainwave patterns and alter brain chemistry can produce happy, calming, or even melancholic moods. This is due to its rhythmic and harmonic properties.

RECOGNIZING SOUND WAVELENGTHS

The fundamental units of the auditory universe are sound frequencies, each of which has a distinct pitch or tone. Hertz (Hz) is the unit of measurement for sound frequency; higher frequencies provide sharper, treble-like sounds, and lower frequencies reflect deeper, bass-like tones. Most sounds that are audible to humans fall between 20 and 20,000 Hz. Our auditory experiences are greatly influenced by sound frequencies, which can have a variety of physiological implications.

Sound frequencies that are not within the range of human hearing have been investigated for possible medicinal uses. Ultrasound is a well-known example of a technology used for medical imaging and therapy that produces high-frequency sound waves that are audible to humans. Several frequencies are employed in sound healing and music therapy to focus on particular facets of well-being. For example, lower frequencies can be utilized to encourage meditation and relaxation, while higher frequencies can be used to energize and focus. Understanding the complex interaction between sound and the human body requires an understanding of sound frequencies.

THE ENERGY CENTERS AND CHAKRAS

Chakras are a component of an Eastern philosophical belief system that is especially prevalent in the context of yoga and meditation. According to popular belief, chakras are energy centers or vortices along the spine, each linked to particular attributes, hues, and frequencies. It is thought that these energy centers control different facets of our mental, emotional, and spiritual health. Even if the idea of chakras may not be supported by science, alternative, and holistic health modalities heavily rely on it.

About chakras, sound and music are frequently utilized to harmonize and balance these energy centers. It is thought that some sound frequencies, which are frequently connected to particular notes in music, can resonate with and affect the chakras, fostering harmony and well-being. Chanting, toning, or listening to particular sounds or mantras that match to the chakras are common methods used in sound therapy and meditation to calm or excite these energy centers. Many people find solace and therapeutic benefit in these practices, even if the scientific basis for chakras and their connection to sound is still up for debate.

The effects of sound on the human body are complex, influencing not just our hearing system but also our emotions, moods, and even energy centers such as chakras. Gaining an understanding of sound frequencies is essential to realizing the distinct effects that various tones and vibrations can have on our health. While certain aspects of sound's influence on the body have a scientific basis, others, like the concept of chakras, are deeply established in belief systems and alternative medical practices. Nonetheless, the relationship between sound and the human body is a rich and fascinating subject of inquiry.

CHAPTER THREE

INSTRUMENTS AND TOOLS

AN OVERVIEW OF SOUND THERAPY INSTRUMENTS

Sound therapy is a holistic approach to healing and relaxation that utilizes various instruments to produce specific vibrations, frequencies, and tones to promote well-being. These instruments are designed to create harmonic, soothing, or resonant sounds that can positively impact one's physical, mental, and emotional state. Some of the most commonly used sound therapy instruments include singing bowls, tuning forks, gongs, crystal bowls, chimes, and drums.

Singing bowls, also known as Tibetan singing bowls or Himalayan singing bowls, are a central component of sound therapy. They are often made of metal alloys and are played by striking or rubbing a mallet around the bowl's rim. The vibrations and harmonious tones they produce can induce deep relaxation and meditation, making them popular choices for stress reduction and mindfulness practices.

Tuning forks are precision instruments that emit specific frequencies when struck. They are used to create precise vibrational frequencies that can be applied to different parts of the body or energy centers (chakras) to stimulate balance and alignment. Tuning forks are commonly used in sound therapy to address specific health and emotional issues.

Gongs, with their wide range of harmonics and frequencies, produce powerful and complex soundscapes. They are often used to clear energy blockages, induce deep relaxation, and promote healing. Crystal bowls, made of pure quartz crystal, produce clear and resonant tones that can have a profound impact on one's energy field and emotional state.

Chimes and wind instruments like flutes and panpipes are used for their calming and grounding qualities, enhancing relaxation and meditation experiences. Drums, including frame drums and hand drums, provide rhythmic and primal beats that can help with stress reduction and achieving altered states of consciousness.

HOW TO CHOOSE THE RIGHT INSTRUMENTS

Selecting the right sound therapy instruments is a personal and sometimes therapeutic journey. When choosing these instruments, it's essential to consider several factors to ensure they align with your specific needs and preferences.

First, consider your purpose for using sound therapy. Are you looking to reduce stress, enhance meditation, or address specific physical or emotional concerns? Different instruments have varying effects, so understanding your objectives will help you choose the most appropriate ones.

Next, evaluate the instrument's sound quality. High-quality instruments produce clear, resonant tones that are vital for effective sound therapy. You can test the instrument's sound in person or listen to recordings if purchasing online.

Consider the materials and craftsmanship of the instrument. Many traditional instruments, like Tibetan singing bowls and crystal bowls, are made by skilled artisans using specific techniques and materials. High-quality materials and craftsmanship can greatly impact the instrument's effectiveness and durability.

Choose instruments that resonate with you on a personal level. The aesthetics, size, and overall feel of the instrument should be pleasing and comfortable to you. Your connection with the instrument can enhance the therapeutic experience.

Budget is also an important factor. Sound therapy instruments come in a wide price range, so it's essential to find instruments that meet your needs without straining your finances.

Lastly, take your time to research and explore different instruments. Experiment with various options and, if possible, consult with experienced sound therapists or practitioners for guidance and recommendations.

HOW TO CARE FOR YOUR SOUND HEALING TOOLS

Proper care of sound healing instruments is essential to maintain their effectiveness and longevity. Here are some general guidelines for caring for these tools:

1. Cleanliness: Regularly clean your instruments to remove dust, dirt, or residue that can affect their sound quality. Use a soft, clean cloth to wipe the surface of metal singing bowls, gongs, and other instruments. Crystal bowls can be gently cleaned with a mild detergent and warm water.

Avoid using abrasive materials that can scratch the surface.

2. Storage: Store your instruments in a safe and dry place to prevent damage or corrosion. Keep them in padded cases or soft cloth bags to protect them from physical harm and environmental factors.

3. Handling: Handle your instruments with care. Avoid dropping or banging them, as this can lead to damage or changes in their vibrational qualities. When using mallets or strikers, apply the right amount of pressure without excessive force.

4. Tuning: Tuning forks may require occasional adjustment or tuning to maintain their precise frequencies. Consult the manufacturer's guidelines or seek professional assistance for tuning if needed.

CHAPTER FOUR

TECHNIQUES AND PRACTICES

SOUND THERAPY IN TRADITIONAL MEDICINE

Sound therapy is a holistic healing practice that has been utilized for centuries in traditional medicine systems across the world. It involves the use of sound vibrations to promote physical, emotional, and spiritual well-being. One of the central principles of sound therapy is the belief that sound has the power to influence the body's energy systems and restore balance. Various techniques and instruments are employed in this therapeutic approach, and they differ based on the culture and tradition in which they are practiced.

SOUND HEALING IN VARIOUS CULTURES

In the realm of sound healing, different cultures have their unique methods and instruments for achieving healing and harmonization. These practices often incorporate a deep connection with nature and spirituality. Native American traditions, for example, emphasize the significance of drumming and chanting. Native American drumming and chanting have been used for centuries to invoke spiritual connection and healing. The rhythmic beat of the drum and the melodic chants are believed to align individuals with the energies of the earth and the spirit world. This not only promotes emotional and mental well-being but also strengthens the bonds within the community.

Tibetan singing bowls are another notable element of sound healing. Originating from Tibetan Buddhism, these bowls are made from a blend of metals and are known for their rich, resonant sound. The vibrations produced by striking or rubbing the bowl's rim are thought to purify the mind, body, and soul. Tibetan singing bowls are used in meditation and healing practices to create a state of deep relaxation and mindfulness. This tradition places great importance on the harmonic frequencies emitted by the bowls as a means to balance the body's chakras and restore harmony.

TIBETAN SINGING BOWLS

Sound healing practices extend beyond the Tibetan tradition. Various cultures worldwide employ their unique instruments and techniques to harness the therapeutic power of sound. From Australian Aboriginal didgeridoos to Hindu mantras and Sanskrit chants, sound healing is deeply embedded in cultural and spiritual traditions. Each culture has its specific rituals and instruments that are believed to facilitate healing, reduce stress, and enhance overall well-being.

Sound therapy is not limited to a particular culture or tradition; it transcends boundaries and is embraced by individuals seeking alternative and complementary forms of healing. The concepts of sound therapy in traditional medicine highlight the profound belief that sound can be a potent tool for healing and transformation, connecting individuals to their inner selves, their communities, and the broader universe. As people continue to explore these practices, they find solace and rejuvenation in the ancient wisdom that sound, in all its forms, has the potential to bring about profound healing and balance in their lives.

CHAPTER FIVE

SOUND THERAPY IN MODERN MEDICINE

Sound therapy, a holistic approach that incorporates diverse sound-based treatments to promote healing and well-being, has gained significance in modern medicine and healthcare. This approach emphasizes the tremendous impact of sound on the human body and mind, and its incorporation into clinical settings offers promising pathways for improving patient outcomes, lowering stress, and promoting general well-being. In this conversation, we explore the applications of sound therapy in hospitals and healthcare, the usage of music therapy in clinical settings, and the necessity of research and evidence-based methods in sound therapy.

SOUND THERAPY IN HOSPITALS AND HEALTHCARE

Sound therapy comprises a broad range of modalities, from music and soundscapes to binaural beats and guided imagery that can be applied in healthcare settings. Hospitals are increasingly recognizing the therapeutic potential of sound to ease pain, reduce anxiety, and promote relaxation. Soundscapes with relaxing natural sounds, such as running water or bird singing, are employed in waiting areas and patient rooms to provide a calming ambiance. In operating rooms, white noise or calming music can assist in alleviating stress and anxiety among both patients and surgical staff. Furthermore, the use of sound therapy in hospitals extends to newborn care units, where lullabies and womb-like sounds can benefit the development of premature infants.

MUSIC THERAPY IN CLINICAL SETTINGS

Music therapy, a well-established kind of sound therapy, involves the use of music treatments to address the physical, emotional, cognitive, and social needs of patients. Music therapists work in clinical settings to construct personalized therapy programs, employing diverse musical techniques, including listening to music, singing, playing instruments, and writing music. These therapies have been particularly successful in mental health facilities, rehabilitation centers, and palliative care units. Music therapy can help patients manage pain, reduce stress and anxiety, improve cognitive function, and promote emotional expressiveness. It is also used to assist persons with autism, Alzheimer's disease, and other neurological diseases.

RESEARCH AND EVIDENCE-BASED PRACTICES

As sound therapy receives respect in modern medicine, the value of research and evidence-based practices cannot be emphasized. Researchers are undertaking studies to evaluate the efficacy of different sound treatment approaches and their effects on patient outcomes. The outcomes of these studies are crucial in directing healthcare providers to apply sound therapy efficiently. For instance, research has shown that music therapy helps lower pain perception during medical operations and enhances the emotional state of cancer patients. Research is also identifying the neurophysiologic mechanisms underpinning the therapeutic effects of sound therapy, shedding light on the complicated link between sound and the human brain.

Sound therapy has become a vital supplement to modern medicine and healthcare. Its applications in hospitals and therapeutic settings are numerous, spanning a vast array of sound-based approaches, with music therapy being a prominent example. Research and evidence-based methods play a critical role in ensuring that sound therapy is applied effectively, delivering patients the benefits of reduced stress, greater well-being, and enhanced medical outcomes. As the awareness of the therapeutic potential of sound therapy continues to improve, its integration into healthcare settings is anticipated to expand, enabling a more holistic and patient-centered approach to medical care.

CHAPTER SIX

CREATING YOUR SOUND HEALING SPACE

SETTING UP A SACRED SPACE

Creating a sound healing space is a significant activity that involves careful consideration of several fundamental elements. One of the key parts is setting up a holy place that generates an environment conducive to healing and transformation. Both the practitioner and the patient can connect with the healing energies and vibrations of sound in this setting, which functions as a sanctuary. Selecting a place that has a spiritual resonance for you is crucial to creating such a space. This could be a special place in your house, a section of your garden, or a section of the outdoors.

Your sacred space's design and aesthetics are very important in establishing the ideal mood. It is best to include items that are symbolic or have particular meaning for you, like sacred geometry, crystals, artwork, or objects that symbolize your spiritual views. This contributes to establishing the energy and intention for the therapeutic work that will be done in this room. To improve the mood and coziness of the space overall, take into account the use of natural materials, gentle lighting, and comfortable seats.

ACOUSTICS AND AMBIENCE

A key factor in determining how successful your sound healing sessions are is the acoustics and ambiance of your space. Being a vibrational medium, sound and its surroundings can have a big impact on how healing is experienced. Consider aspects like room dimensions, design, and building materials to maximize the acoustics in your area. For sound healing work, rooms with good reverberation where sound can linger and harmonize are frequently chosen.

To manage sound reflections and produce a more harmonious audio environment, use acoustic treatments like wall hangings, drapes, or rugs. It also matters the instruments you use and where you put them in the room. Take into account how the acoustics of the room affect the sounds produced by crystal bowls, gongs, Tibetan singing bowls, and other instruments.

Temperature and lighting play a major role in ambiance. While keeping the temperature suitable guarantees that your clients can unwind completely during the session, soft, warm lighting can help create a calming ambiance. An atmosphere that is calmer and more immersive can also be achieved by aromatherapy techniques like using incense or essential oils. Together, these components improve the whole experience, making it cozier and more restorative.

GETTING READY FOR HEALING SESSIONS

The effectiveness of your healing sessions as a sound healer depends greatly on your state of being. You will need to prepare yourself mentally, physically, and spiritually for these sessions. It's crucial to first develop an inner sense of balance and tranquility. This could be deep breathing techniques, meditation, or any other self-centered and grounding activity. Being present for your clients requires purging distractions and fears from your head.

It's also critical to preserve your own physical and mental well-being. Maintaining a regular self-care regimen that includes healthy eating, exercise, and enough sleep enhances your general well-being. Since sound healing is a physically demanding technique, giving your sessions their best chance will depend on your physical state.

Think about your aims and mindset as well. Have an honest intention to assist healing and transformation in every session and approach it with a pure heart. Your voice and energy will carry this sense of purpose, giving your clients a more potent and therapeutic experience.

Establishing a sacred space that is aesthetically and energetically pleasant is a necessary step in developing a sound healing area. Acoustics and atmosphere are crucial considerations because they have a big influence on how productive your sessions are. Finally, to provide your clients with the finest experience possible, you must prepare yourself for healing sessions by concentrating on your intention, mindset, and physical and mental well-being. Your sound healing area becomes a haven of healing and transformation when all these elements come together.

CHAPTER SEVEN

APPLICATIONS OF SOUND THERAPY

UTILIZING SOUND THERAPY TO REDUCE STRESS

A holistic approach, sound therapy uses sound's calming and stress-relieving properties to improve people's general well-being. This ancient practice, which has been employed for millennia in many different cultures worldwide, is based on the idea that music has the power to affect both our mental and physical states. We'll talk about how sound therapy may be used to reduce stress, how sound can be used for relaxation and meditation, how to breathe, and how sound is related to mindfulness.

In contemporary medicine, sound therapy is becoming more and more used as an alternative and supplemental treatment for stress reduction. Stress and anxiety can be reduced by listening to relaxing music and nature sounds recorded on instruments like singing bowls, tuning forks, wind chimes, and even recorded nature sounds. The body's relaxation response can be triggered and stress hormones like cortisol can be lessened by these noises' capacity to entrain brainwaves and induce a deep state of relaxation.

RELAXATION WITH SOUND MEDITATION

Relaxation and sound meditation are essential parts of sound therapy. People usually lie down or sit comfortably during a sound meditation session and let the sounds wash over them. Deeply relaxing meditations can be facilitated by the resonance frequencies and vibrations produced by musical instruments. For people who find it difficult to focus during typical meditation sessions, sound meditation can be particularly beneficial because it offers a focal point to help focus the mind and minimize distractions.

BREATHING METHODOLOGIES

Sessions of sound therapy are often accompanied by breathing exercises. Together with the therapeutic sounds, controlled and attentive breathing exercises can help promote relaxation and lower stress levels. As the sound vibrations align with deep, regular breathing, tension is released and a sense of calm is fostered. The combination of sound and breath can strengthen the mind-body bond and help people become more resilient to challenges in daily life.

SILENCE AND INTENTIONALITY

In sound therapy, sound and mindfulness are closely related concepts. Being mindful entails giving the current moment your undivided attention. By encouraging people to concentrate their consciousness on the sounds they are experiencing, sound therapy promotes this mindfulness. Engaging in attentive listening, observing the subtleties of the sounds, and fully submerging oneself in their vibrations can serve as an effective mindfulness practice. This exercise fosters a more centered and grounded state of mind, increases self-awareness, and strengthens one's connection to the environment.

Sound therapy provides a flexible and successful method for mindfulness, relaxation, and stress reduction. Deep relaxation can be attained by participants in sound therapy sessions thanks to the relaxing sounds and vibrations that reduce stress and anxiety. The effects of sound therapy can be increased by combining sound meditation with controlled breathing exercises, which can improve mental and emotional health. The practice is also in line with the tenets of mindfulness since it promotes complete present-moment awareness, which increases self-awareness and inner serenity.

CHAPTER EIGHT

VIBRANT SOUND THERAPY FOR PHYSICAL RECOVERY

PAIN CONTROL USING SOUND

Sound therapy, sometimes referred to as sound healing, is becoming more widely accepted as a complementary pain management technique. It is an invaluable tool for people recovering from accidents or chronic pain since it uses sound frequencies to facilitate both physical and mental healing. The fundamental tenet of sound therapy for pain relief is that sound waves have the power to affect the body's innate ability to heal itself. These vibrations have the potential to enhance general well-being and lessen pain and discomfort.

The idea that imbalances in the body's energy systems are frequently the cause of pain is one of the core tenets of sound therapy for pain treatment. Certain frequencies of sound can aid in reestablishing this equilibrium, which will relieve pain. In sound therapy sessions, instruments like Tibetan singing bowls, tuning forks, and crystal bowls are frequently used. These instruments have a unique frequency range that when played, resonates with the body's energy centers, or chakras, easing tension and discomfort. These devices produce deep-tissue vibrations that induce relaxation and ease tense muscles, which are frequently linked to physical discomfort.

Additionally, endorphins the body's natural analgesics can be released in response to sound treatment, which enhances well-being and lessens pain perception. When used in conjunction with other therapies, this natural approach to pain management can be very beneficial for people with arthritis, fibromyalgia, or chronic pain.

HARMONIOUS HEALING

One of the main ideas of sound therapy for physical healing is vibrational healing. Its foundation is the idea that every living thing, including the human body, has a distinct vibrational frequency. A condition of health and well-being is attained when the body vibrates in unison. Disturbances or imbalances in these vibrations, however, might result in mental and physical illnesses.

The idea behind sound therapy is that the body's natural vibrational frequencies can interact with outside sound waves to bring about a state of equilibrium. It is said that certain instruments and music frequencies resonate with particular energy centers and parts of the body, balancing the vibrations and resolving health problems. In this situation, the "instrument" is the body, and the objective is to tune it for maximum health.

This idea is comparable to tuning a musical instrument to produce harmonious sounds.

A range of instruments and methods are employed by sound therapists to promote vibrational healing. To generate particular frequencies that resonate with the body's energy centers, people frequently use singing bowls, gongs, and voice toning. The goal of the therapy is to help the body heal physically by encouraging it to return to its natural state of balance by concentrating on these frequencies.

THE IMMUNE SYSTEM AND SOUND

In the realm of holistic healthcare, there is growing interest in the connection between sound treatment and the immune system. The immune system is essential for defending the body against illnesses and infections. People who have weakened or compromised immune systems are more prone to disease. More and more research is showing that sound therapy helps strengthen the body's defenses by lowering stress and encouraging relaxation, both of which can have a favorable impact on the immune system.

One important thing that can compromise the immune system is stress. Stress hormones like cortisol, when persistently increased, can inhibit immunological function. Chronic stress can cause the release of these hormones. Stress levels can be reduced by sound therapy by fostering a feeling of profound relaxation and peace. This could therefore result in a reduction in cortisol production and an improvement in immune system performance.

In addition to relieving pain, sound therapy can also increase the release of endorphins, which have antidepressant and mood-boosting properties. Improved immune function is linked to a happy emotional state. Furthermore, sound therapy's vibrational component is thought to promote the body's energy flow, enhancing general health and fortifying the immune system.

Sound therapy for physical healing provides an all-encompassing strategy for immune system support, vibrational healing, and pain control. It attempts to relieve pain, improve general wellness, and bring the body's energy systems back into balance by utilizing the power of sound frequencies. As the advantages of sound treatment are still being investigated, this area of holistic medicine is both intriguing and exciting.

CHAPTER NINE

SOUND HEALING FOR MENTAL AND EMOTIONAL HEALTH

SOUND AND EMOTIONAL RELEASE

Using the power of sound to enhance emotional and mental well-being, sound therapy—also known as sound healing or sound meditation—is a holistic approach. It is predicated on the idea that sound waves can profoundly affect our emotions, allowing us to let go of repressed emotions and discover inner equilibrium. This therapeutic approach combines sound with emotional discharge.

Singing bowls, gongs, chimes, drums, and tuning forks are just a few of the instruments used by sound therapy practitioners to produce resonant, harmonic tones that can resonate deep into the body and psyche. People can have a cathartic experience by letting go of stress and emotional blocks with the aid of these sounds. Known as "feel-good" hormones, endorphins are released when the body's natural relaxation response is stimulated by the vibrations produced during a sound therapy session. People can release negative emotions, stress, and anxiety through this method, which helps with emotional release.

ANXIETY AND DEPRESSION WITH SOUND THERAPY

Anxiety and depression are common mental health issues that can be difficult to treat. As an alternative to traditional therapies for these ailments, sound therapy has gained popularity since it provides a special means of promoting mental health and emotional relaxation.

People undergoing sound therapy for anxiety and depression are exposed to particular sound frequencies and patterns, which have the potential to calm the mind and reduce symptoms. The physiological and psychological signs of worry, such as accelerated heart rate and racing thoughts, can be lessened with the use of sound therapy's soothing and harmonizing tones. Sound therapy can reduce anxiety symptoms and promote emotional peace by rewiring the brain to a more relaxed state.

Sound therapy can be an effective means of fostering happy feelings in those suffering from depression. Those who are suffering from depression symptoms may find that the soft, resonating sounds uplift them and give them a sense of inner calm. Additionally, sound therapy can help redirect attention from negative thought patterns and promote a more optimistic outlook.

NURTURING PLEASANT EMOTIONS

Sound therapy is important for fostering pleasant emotions as well as for reducing negative ones. In sound therapy, specific vibrations and frequencies are employed to establish a feeling of balance and harmony inside the patient's emotional field.

The encouragement of relaxation and stress reduction is one of the main ways sound therapy fosters happy feelings. Positive feelings rise to the surface naturally when tension fades. Joy, satisfaction, and calm can be evoked during a sound therapy session by the relaxing noises. These feelings might last long after the session is complete, which enhances general well-being.

Additionally, sound therapy can support the development of mindfulness and self-awareness. People can better comprehend their emotions and increase their ability to cultivate happy feelings by making a connection with the sounds and vibrations of the present moment. A happier and more resilient emotional state may result from this enhanced awareness.

Sound therapy is an effective and adaptable strategy for promoting emotional and mental health.

CHAPTER TEN

SUPERIOR SOUND THERAPY

VIBRATIONAL HEALING AND ENERGY MEDICINE

A comprehensive approach, sound therapy uses vibrations and sound waves to enhance mental, emotional, and physical health. Sound therapy is an important part of energy medicine because it makes use of the idea that everything in the universe, including our bodies, vibrates at a particular frequency. This idea is the foundation of sound therapy, which holds that the body's energy systems may be brought back into harmony and balance by employing sound and particular frequencies. Its basis is the idea that music has the power to affect the body's energy fields, resulting in enhanced general health and vigor.

HARMONY WITH THE CHAKRAS

The connection between sound treatment and the chakras is an important feature. Energy centers called chakras are found along the spine and are thought to be vital to our general health and well-being. There is a particular hue, tone, and vibrational frequency linked to each chakra. To stimulate and balance the chakras, practitioners of sound therapy employ a variety of sound instruments, including tuning forks, singing bowls, and chanting. By using particular frequencies and sounds, practitioners hope to remove blockages and encourage the free flow of energy through these energy centers, which can have a significant effect on one's physical and emotional health. For instance, the root chakra is connected to the color red and the sound "Lam."

CRYSTAL HEALING AND SOUND

Another intriguing idea in sound therapy is sound healing using crystals. Since ancient times, people have utilized crystals, which are recognized for their distinctive vibrational frequencies, to encourage balance and healing. Crystals can intensify the sound's therapeutic effects when used in conjunction with sound therapy. Sound healing approaches have seen a rise in the popularity of crystal singing bowls in particular. Every crystal bowl has a distinct chakra associated with it and emits a pure tone when struck. The crystal singing bowls' vibrations resonate with the body's energy, assisting in stress relief, imbalance restoration, and obstruction clearing. Participants in sound therapy sessions may enjoy a profoundly calming and therapeutic atmosphere thanks to the sound and crystal combination.

FRAGRANCE AND AUDIO

Sound and aromatherapy are frequently used to improve the therapeutic process overall. Essential oils, which come from a variety of plants and each have special medicinal qualities, are used in aromatherapy. Essential oils can enhance the vibrational therapeutic properties of sound when they are applied topically or diffused during a sound therapy session. The individual's demands, such as enhancing energy, lowering worry, or encouraging relaxation, are taken into consideration while selecting essential oils. Combining aromatherapy and sound therapy can result in a multisensory experience that addresses emotional and psychological well-being in addition to the energetic aspects of healing.

CHAPTER ELEVEN

BOTH MEDITATION AND SOUND THERAPY

For attaining mental and emotional equilibrium, improving mindfulness, and fostering general well-being, sound therapy, and meditation are effective strategies. The practice of incorporating sound into meditation has grown in popularity recently since it can enhance the meditative experience and provide several advantages for those who practice it. Here, sound is employed to enhance conventional meditation techniques and assist practitioners in reaching a deeper level of inner peace and relaxation.

INCLUDING MUSIC IN YOUR MEDITATION

There are several ways to incorporate sound into meditation, including gongs, singing bowls, chanting, and background noise. These noises can help people achieve a higher level of awareness during meditation by guiding and supporting the process. By adding sound, meditation becomes a multisensory experience that stimulates the body and the mind, resulting in a deeper inner connection.

A typical usage of sound elements in meditation is mantras and affirmations. During meditation, one might use mantras—sacred words, phrases, or sounds—to help focus the mind and improve attention. These monotonous noises provide a calming pattern that encourages relaxation and aids in distracting attention. For instance, the "Om" mantra is commonly employed in many forms of meditation because it is thought to symbolize the sound of the universe and help the practitioner become more in tune with the universe.

AFFIRMATIONS & MANTRAS

Conversely, affirmations are uplifting words or sentiments that are repeated during meditation to foster a more upbeat outlook and promote personal development. These affirmations can be tailored to target particular objectives or desires, such as stress reduction, confidence building, or thankfulness cultivation. While meditation, repeating affirmations can help rewire the subconscious and foster a more positive attitude toward life.

PRODUCING RESTORATIVE SOUNDSCAPES

Another method of using sound in meditation is to create therapeutic soundscapes. Immersion aural settings called "soundscapes" are intentionally created to promote calm and ease the transition into meditation. They frequently blend instrumental or electronic music with ambient noises like wind, water, and birdsong to create a calming symphony. People can escape the strains of everyday life and lose themselves in a serene and soothing audio world by using soundscapes to take them to a new mental dimension.

Soundscapes can be combined with other sound elements, such as mantras or affirmations, or used alone as a meditation technique. They offer a multisensory experience that helps lower blood pressure, lessen anxiety, and improve mental clarity. Making healing soundscapes can be a very powerful approach to improving your meditation practice, regardless of your preference for the sound of waves crashing on the shore, soft leaves rustling in a forest, or the resonance of crystal singing bowls.

Sound therapy and meditation are complementary holistic modalities that can work well together. Mantras, affirmations, and therapeutic soundscapes can all be used to include sound in meditation, which can enhance your practice and have several psychological, emotional, and physical advantages.

CHAPTEER TWELVE

USING SOUND THERAPY TO TRANSFORM YOURSELF

SELF-REPAIR METHODS

Self-healing methods are a common component of sound therapy for personal transformation. These methods are predicated on the notion that, in the correct circumstances, our bodies and brains possess the innate capacity to self-heal. Through the use of various sonic frequencies, including music, singing bowls, and even human voice, sound therapy can activate the body's natural healing processes. This type of therapy helps people access their inherent healing capacity while promoting calm and lowering stress.

Meditation is one of the main self-healing methods utilized in sound therapy. When combined with particular sound frequencies, meditation helps people de-stress, calm down, and achieve a deep level of relaxation. In this condition, the body can make use of its natural healing capacities, fostering mental, emotional, and physical health. Incorporating breathing exercises and mindfulness techniques into sound therapy practices is a common way to improve the capacity for self-healing.

EXPRESSION AND TONE

The idea of manifestation the process of making one's reality by directing one's thoughts, intentions, and energy toward particular objectives or desires is frequently linked to sound therapy. Sound can manifest because it can affect our feelings, thoughts, and vibrational energy. Sound waves have the power to align with our intents and objectives, supporting the manifestation of those goals.

Practitioners of sound therapy hold that people can raise their vibrational frequency to a point where they are more responsive to the energies that attract their wishes by employing sound as a manifestation technique. In sound therapy sessions, mantras, affirmations, and intention-setting are frequently used techniques. To enhance the manifestation process, these are mixed with melodious instruments or vocalization sounds. People try to make the reality they want by using sound to cultivate a happy and focused mindset.

THE PATH TO COMPLETENESS

One of the main ideas of sound therapy for personal development is the road to wholeness. It is based on the notion that people are capable of healing, transforming, and integrating all facets of who they are—physical, emotional, and spiritual. To assist people in connecting with their true essence and accessing their inner resources, sound therapy acts as a guide and catalyst for this journey.

Sound therapy acts as a bridge to promote balance and harmony inside an individual during their path toward completeness. Through the use of different sound frequencies and healing procedures, people are said to be able to let go of past traumas, get past emotional obstacles, and feel whole. Deep introspection, self-reflection, and self-discovery are frequently part of this path.

Furthermore, the path to wholeness is a never-ending process of self-realization and evolution rather than a straight line. It is about realizing the connection between the mind, body, and spirit and accepting oneself as one truly is. By establishing a safe and encouraging environment for personal growth, assisting people in overcoming obstacles, and promoting a sense of inner serenity and harmony, sound therapy supports this journey.

CHAPTER THIRTEEN

MORAL DETERMINATIONS

ETHICAL BEHAVIOR IN SOUND TREATMENT

To give clients responsible and effective care, ethical practice in sound therapy is crucial. Utilizing different sound-based methods to enhance relaxation, healing, and general well-being, such as singing bowls, tuning forks, or music, is known as sound therapy. To preserve the trust, safety, and efficacy of the therapy, ethical considerations must be prioritized in this therapeutic method.

THE SIGNIFICANCE OF KNOWLEDGEABLE CONSENT

Consent that has been informed is crucial in any therapeutic setting. This idea is the same in sound treatment. It is implied by informed consent that clients have a right to be fully informed about the nature of sound therapy, its possible advantages, and any risks or discomforts that may be related to the treatment. The aims and goals of the therapy, as well as the anticipated length and frequency of sessions, must be discussed by the therapists. In addition, clients must be given the chance to inquire and give their consent voluntarily, free from any kind of compulsion. Establishing transparent and truthful communication fosters trust and gives patients the ability to make knowledgeable decisions about their care.

BOUNDARIES AND CONFIDENTIALITY

Sound therapy's ethical pillars are confidentiality and boundaries. When discussing their ideas, feelings, and experiences with their therapists, clients need to feel comfortable and safe doing so. Since sound therapy frequently explores deeply ingrained emotions, secrecy guarantees that clients can express themselves honestly without worrying about being judged or having their private information revealed. Therapists have an ethical duty to respect their clients' privacy and only divulge information to outside parties with the client's express permission and when it is necessary for the client's well-being.

Furthermore, sound therapy places a premium on upholding appropriate and transparent limits. To distinguish themselves from friends or family, therapists need to set professional boundaries. These limits are required to avoid any dual partnerships that can jeopardize the therapeutic exchange. To provide a secure and predictable atmosphere where the emphasis is kept on the client's well-being and personal development, clients must be aware of what to expect from the therapist in terms of conduct and activities.

KEEPING CUSTOMERS SAFE

Ensuring client safety is a crucial ethical responsibility in sound therapy. To reduce the possibility of injury, therapists need to be skilled and knowledgeable in their work. This entails having the appropriate understanding of sound treatment methods, tools, and possible outcomes. To make sure that treatment is suitable and safe for their clients, therapists should also routinely evaluate their client's mental and physical conditions. The therapist should always put the client's needs first and be ready to modify or stop therapy if a client exhibits symptoms of discomfort or distress during a session.